THE SENSE ABOUT MADNESS

THE SENSE ABOUT MADNESS:

A Raw Look at Child Abuse, Sexual Violence, and Mental Illness

Alyssa K. Vine-Hodge

Copyright 2015 by Alyssa K. Vine-Hodge
ISBN 978-0-692-48226-1

Front Cover Photo by John Vine-Hodge
Back Cover Photo by Tessa Maxine Photography

This story reflects the author's true experiences. Individuals written about gave consent, or names, dates, and event locations were purposefully omitted so as to respect privacy and protect identity.

This book is dedicated to:

Those who are fighting through their pain, and to those who burn with a passion to lift up all oppressed, advocating for justice and change.

A special thanks to:

Myra Schwartz, for looking at the book with an editorial eye and inspiring me to put it out there.

My brother Josh Vine and my friend Amanda Pokrzywa, for reading the content in its most raw form and giving me the encouragement to continue.

Book Overview

Foreword

Introduction: How this Book Happened

The Writing Process

****

Chapter One: Touching Hell: *Waking up insane and finding myself committed*

When the wrinkles of the mind unravel, sanity becomes a maze. Past deceptions become the present truth. There are no more lines between darkness and light, only chaos.

Chapter Two: A Letter Unsent

What do we do when the bad guys get away with it? When they win? Sometimes justice becomes something we have to create within ourselves. When justice fails to be delivered on our behalf, we must search for sweetness in the bitter sting.

Chapter Three: The Puzzle of a Shattered Psyche

A puzzle can be quite frustrating and overwhelming until the image starts to emerge. When life shatters us, we will always have cracks, but even in brokenness, there is beauty and meaning.

****

Epilogue

About the Author

Foreword

I am the licensed, professional counselor that is frequently included in this awesome narrative you are about to read. I am proud of the author and her desire to help others, as people abused or as abuser, to heal. This story does matter a lot.

The reactions to this story will be varied. For some, the images will be too tough to imagine while others may find the solution to be as simple as, "Get over it!!" For some, the healing will seem incomplete. And some may see the connection with God as inconsistent with their spiritual belief system.

This is a living story that will continue to bring pain, resolve, and some healing. I pray that God will enter each such story to bring a lasting sense of value to the abused victim and to each abuser the desire to get help to stop their abuse.

Read this story with an open heart. Seek ways to help those among you who have these deep wounds and/or scars. The best way most can help is to hear the person's story—believe it is perspectively true—know that correcting the perspective is difficult, if possible—admire the tenacity to keep healing—support the person with the tough history so they can live life with some laughter, some tears, some sleepless nights, some seemingly wasted days, and not feel condemned to a life full of torment and rejection.

The pain is not their fault. The healing process is their responsibility to enter. The life so supported will benefit all who give.

—**Bill Buck**
Relationship Counselor, Raleigh, NC

Introduction: How this Book Happened

"The Sense about Madness" is the second most important book I've ever written. The first was a story called "Puppy Love" that I wrote when I was a five-year-old girl. My mom helped me put it together, bind it in a homemade hard copy and "publish" it with my name on the front cover. She was an elementary school teacher and her favorite subject to teach was creative writing. She loved inspiring children to express themselves through writing and bask in the satisfaction of "publishing" it, seeing their names on the front of something they'd written. So naturally, as my mom, she enjoyed doing the same for me.

"Puppy Love" was the story of my personal pain...the pain of finding a lost puppy, loving it so much for one day, and then having to give it back to the original owner and say good-bye. This was the saddest day of my little kindergarten life.

"*How* can you make me give this puppy away, mom?"

"I'm not *making* you give it away, honey. We are giving it back to the person it belongs to. It's lost."

"No. It's not lost. It *wanted* to come over to our house and be my friend! See how much it loves me?"

"Come here, Alyssa. We're going to sit down and you are going to write a story about it. You can tell me everything you feel about this puppy. You can illustrate it too. I'll help you make a nice hard cover for it and we'll publish it and put your name on the front. I know you are sad today, but once you write this story you will always have something special to keep and remember how much you love this puppy."

To put it in adult language, I was pretty pissed at my mom. I had never been pushed to such an emotional edge. I didn't have the vocabulary to go with my feelings then, but I was experiencing utter frustration, loss, loneliness, and grief. I had tried to explain to my mom that I was the saddest I had ever been in my whole life and she said, "Write a book about it." It felt like chastisement, like she really didn't get it, and was just faking sympathy.

Over the years, I did go back and look at that book several times. I thought it was cute and sad. And, it made me laugh to see it. I would tease my mom sometimes, still whining just for fun, "Mom, I still don't understand how you could make me give that puppy away and tell me to write about it." "Because, we *knew* who the owner was, honey." "Oh, okay." I'm grown up now, so the logic makes sense.

I never really understood though, until recently, just how powerful a gift my mom had actually given to me that day. She *sat with me* and *helped* me compose my book. She *listened* to my pain. She *showed* me that even when we can't change our circumstances, our feelings are still worth expressing. The written word has power. She *taught* me that there is purpose in creating something out of my pain — that books are like treasures, and that when your name appears on the front cover, it's an accomplishment to feel proud of.

Since that day over 30 years ago, writing when I was hurting has been something I've always done. I wouldn't just write my own pain, but I would write stories and poems about the pain I saw in the world around me…every once in a while writing about something happy just to mix it up.

Mostly, I would keep the writings to myself, like a private journal where I could write my darkest secrets. Alone, and with my pen, I felt the freedom to let out whatever was bottled inside. But revealing my words to anyone proved difficult. What if people judge what I say? What if my words disappoint them, make them frightened, or angry?

"The Sense about Madness" is my debut. I had a closet that I needed to come out of—a closet full of secrets and shame. So dark and terrifying was my closet, I thought if I came out of it I might die. I almost did. I only gained the courage to open the door when continuing to live in my closet became as frightening as dying in it. And it is only because of the people who have loved me that I've had the strength to survive. I needed the science of medicine, I needed the God of the universe, every angel and heavenly host, all the ones who had gone before me, every earthly prayer ever uttered over my life, every positive thought and kind word, every smile ever flashed in my direction, every embrace I've ever felt, every family member, and every friend to help me crawl through that door.

So, this book is first and foremost an enormous act of self-love, a task I'm still working very hard at learning how to do. It is my first time exposing certain truths about myself without wrapping everything up neatly in an apology. And secondly, it is my "thank you," my expression of gratitude for the gift of survival. Lastly, it is a call to action that we may speak boldly in a communal embrace of support for those who feel bound in the silence of pain.

It is my hope that even though the material is dark, glimmers of hope may shine through, illuminating the human spirit.

The Writing Process

This book was written over a five year period, after I was hospitalized for a psychotic breakdown that occurred when I was in my early thirties. I was diagnosed with Bipolar I Disorder and Post Traumatic Stress Disorder, and through counseling, began to work through surfacing memories of childhood sexual abuse.

This book began as a compilation of journal entries, poems, and letters that I wrote throughout the recovery process. The book reflects this process, and the information is not always chronological. I tell my story as I speak, so phrases that may be grammatically incorrect are intentional.

Recovery is ongoing. I am not "all better now." But I have gotten to a place of healing where I feel the information is shareable. Having a completed body of work on my book shelf also helps me to feel a healthy sense of completion and control over the senseless things that happened in my life.

Much thought went into deciding which parts of my writing would be part of the book and how to organize everything. At first, I wanted to share every detail about the abuse that happened to me. But that option left me with questions. Will I need to use a pen name? Will someone doubt my personal truth and attack me? I wrote many unsent cathartic letters: Letters to the family of the abuser, letters to the editor, the town council, my parents, and on and on. Ultimately, I chose to only include one in the book (found in Chapter 2)—the letter I wrote to my abuser, who is now deceased.

I fully understand the need survivors have for sharing every horrific detail. And I support that need to be heard.

Every person who has been victimized should have the right to be heard—FULLY.

As I worked through my process, the message I needed to get out evolved. It became less about the specific details of the abuse and my feelings and more about the overall destructive nature of abuse, my path of confrontation, and my desire to provoke and inspire action.

I also felt that I did not want to share my story until I got to a point where I was able to laugh at it, at least in part. This does not mean I laugh at abuse. But for me comedy is a means of survival, and to find flickers of moments that I could laugh at in my times of darkness is what holds me intact.

In sharing my book with a few people prior to publication, some still found it quite dark, with the comedic elements hard to find. Others found the material to be "moving," "brave," and "hopeful." I hope that whatever adjective you as the reader might ascribe to the book, my words will leave something of substance that ignites understanding and action.

I'm not proud enough to think I've written anything here which hasn't been said before. But I'm convinced enough that the same words need to be said over and over again, until they wash over humankind like waves, cleansing us of the toxicity of abuse, and liberating every person in its grip.

Chapter One: Touching Hell: *Waking up insane and finding myself committed*

"Even when you're crazy, you're still kind of cute."

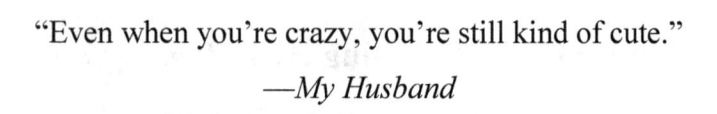

—My Husband

The Car Ride

Staring straight ahead, I nervously glance over at my husband from time to time as he drives along the interstate. His pensive expression, the exhaustion and frustration on his face, looks so aggressive. I just know at any point he is about to turn into a monster I've seen before and hurt me. I can feel the warm urine running down my legs, soaking my clothes, and pooling underneath me in the passenger seat. I wonder if he notices that I just peed right here beside him in the car.

I sit here in my silent anguish. I hear thousands of mice behind me in the back seat scurrying and squealing. I turn around to look, realizing they are not really there. We drive past a house on a hill. I hear the screams of tortured animals coming from the house. My husband doesn't seem to notice. I keep asking him for more water. He seems agitated at my requests. For some reason, I just can't drink enough to quench my thirst and to feel cleansed.

I know I'm going crazy again and I'll eventually need to get to a hospital. He pulls off at an exit to see if I need to use the bathroom. I can feel myself trembling. This is it. It's over. I can sense him about to snap at any second. I don't want to see that monster. I can't bear it. In a final effort to save myself from certain demise, I jump into his lap and burst into tears pleading, "Please don't murder me! Please don't murder me!"

At this, I can see his expression soften. He puts his arms around me and looks into my eyes. "You know me," he sweetly speaks. "I'm not going to murder you. I would never hurt you." I'm not sure if I can fully trust him, but I choose to. I embrace him, clinging to him, my teary face pressed into his shoulder. I feel my body relax with the knowledge that his words are true. I do know him. He's not going to hurt me after all. I want him to hold me forever so that the panic won't return.

"Do you think you can walk into the McDonald's now and go to the bathroom...*by yourself,* Alyssa?" I want to show him that I'm strong...that I won't let him lose me to insanity.

I want it so much that it gives me the strength to say yes. So I open the car door and walk up the hill across the parking lot. I can do this. And I do.

I can't stop myself from smiling with pride along the way. I'm *really* doing it. To my surprise, everyone who makes eye contact with me in the restaurant smiles back. Their gazes feel long, sincere, and comforting. It feels like pure love and acceptance. I wonder if it really is, or if they're smiling because they see a crazy girl who peed her pants. I choose to stay with the feeling of the former, basking in all the positive energy of these people I'll never see again. I smile all the way back to the car. It's funny that this walk to the McDonald's bathroom is probably the life accomplishment that I'm most proud of.

Twisted Mind

I have kaleidoscope eyes and a twisted mind that lies behind. I see a distorted reality…colors in motion, parts of a whole…beauty out of reach then too close for me to handle.

At rare times, the motion stops and I see reality comfortably. But I'm told it isn't true. "Euphoria is mania," the textbooks say. And I know they're right, because no matter where I seem to stand in heaven, the door to hell is always still right next to me. It feels peaceful to me now though. Love is all around and all of creation seems to hum the right tune. Nothing alarms and nothing doesn't belong. Fear does not exist here. I'll enjoy this for as long as it lasts.

When the motion starts again, anxiety comes because all the comfort around me starts twisting and turning. This is when the terror sets in. I see demons in the night. My mind plays tricks on me by day. Expressions, questions, statements, and touches all confuse me and seem to take pleasure in the fact that I am afraid.

It feels like I'm either floating away or being pressed down. At times the terror paralyzes me. I see the black presence hovering right over my body. It's pressing me down so I can't move or think. It feels like something right from the pit of hell. It wants to kill me. It has the power to. I can only pray one word over and over again as I wait for the presence to finally lift. I thank God for pulling it off of me, when it finally does. I still tremble even though it's gone.

What haunts me now is the blackness behind my eyes, the memories I can't fully recall. My young eyes split in two directions, confusion to my left, a prize reward to my right. I can't recall with certainty the words, explanation, or participation. I only know what it felt like, or rather feels like still.

Now my body shuts down. I go blind in my left eye. My right eye turns faster and faster. I can't find what I need…who I need. Here comes the fight for my sanity. There is no escape. This is the part of the battle I must fight alone. I pray that I can make it 'til morning and that my eyes will readjust.

I lay in my bed holding on for dear life. My husband is sleeping so peacefully beside me. I move close to him and put my head and left hand on his back. If I lay here and just feel him breathing, I'll know that I'm alive…safe like a little baby in the womb, connected to her mother's breath and heartbeat. I begin to relax and breathe peacefully too for a moment.

But now I'm beginning to lose myself. I can't feel myself breathing anymore. *Oh my God I'm dying!* "*Come back!*" I tell myself. "*Okay. Okay, I'm still here. I'm still touching my husband. Maybe I should focus on my own breath instead of his."* So I do. Peace returns for a minute. *Yes, I'm breathing. I'm alive.*

But as I concentrate on my breath, I start to lose the sensation of his. I cease to feel the life in his body. He feels clammy. Dead. The panic returns. "*Oh my God, he's dead!*" When I feel him breathe, I cease to feel the life in myself. When I feel myself breathe, I cease to feel the life in him. "*Please God make this pendulum stop swinging!*"

I can no longer negotiate the peaceful balance anymore, that perfect point of connection where I can feel us both alive and breathing. I'm utterly petrified. Terror has invaded every cell in my body. This is when I wake my husband up and whisper, "I need to get to a hospital now please, or I'm not gonna be able to make it."

The Emergency Room

The lights are so bright in here. The noises are chaotic. Nurses shuffle in and out asking me questions. My husband and my parents take turns in the room standing at my side. I sure wish my dog could be here with me too.

I am loud. I shout absurdities, at times bringing myself to fits of laughter. I'm frightened too. Pieces of past traumas are starting to come out. "Did someone touch you?" my mom asks, referring to my childhood. "I don't think so…but I think I might have seen something." It will take me two more years to remember what really happened.

My mom explains that I'm laying on a machine and that I'm about to get a brain scan. My body hurts. I lift my head up to look down at myself laying here in the hospital gown. I pull it open to see what's hurting. I ask my mom why the whole right side of my body is severely black and blue. Seeing it scares me.

"I think it happened at your house when the EMS came to get you honey." Oh yeah. I remember that now. Six people stood around me. I got scared when they laughed at me. I threw a glass of water in that lady's face. I kicked the tall man. He threw me to my kitchen floor. They all pinned me down as someone stuck the tranquilizer needle in my arm. I fought, I cried, I yelled out to my husband to make them stop. It makes sense to me now that I'm black and blue. So I look up at my mom's face, and I nod. I'm so glad she's here with me. My dad too. I need him here.

I'm worried though that I may have hurt my husband's feelings with my raging outbursts. I'm worried that his testicles might throb forever from when I attacked him, thinking he was demon possessed. He was so sweet to me. He let me hurt him and he never hurt me back. He let me do so many things. He cried with me. He held me. He loves me so much that he waited for me to say I needed help when he could have made the decision for me. I have no idea that he hid all the knives in our house, just in case. I feel guilty for scaring him so much, but I can't stop myself. I sure hope they find out what is wrong with me.

The brain scan comes back clear—no tumor. I know I'm being sent somewhere for more help. But I don't realize that I'll be locked away.

The Psych Ward

It's late at night, or early morning. I really don't know what time it is, just that it's dark. Someone from admissions hands me a piece of paper and asks me to sign it. I sign the name of a dead person that I admire, the female comedian Gilda Radner. I don't want to sign my real name because I can't understand what the paper says. I want to make sure I'm not signing my life away. I won't know 'til afterwards that it didn't matter. I had already been committed.

That means my husband can't get me out of here now even if wants to. The people in the white coats have all the power now. I can't leave until they say I can. What if they never do?

"Please don't use restraints on her," my mom asks the staff. "She seems to be doing fine when she is approached gently and kindly." I'm grateful I have a mom that thinks to ask them that.

My family has to leave me now. I'm all on my own, left to negotiate a foreign hallway, interactions with other patients, and medical personnel. I don't know where I am, what to do, or who to trust yet. I won't even remember most of this first week.

I am breaking all the rules without knowing it. The staff members scold me. "You *know* what time telephone hours are. You are smart. Go read all the rules on the wall." They don't seem to understand that I'm so crazy I can't read right now. Words on paper don't make sense. And even when I do grasp the rules, I forget them a few minutes later. All my energy is focused on survival. They don't understand how hard I'm really trying.

I stand at the medication window, waiting to find out when I can have my anxiety medicine. I need it so badly. "You can always tell who the drug addicts are. They're the ones who go up to the window every ten minutes." I turn around to see two staff members snickering at me. "I'm not here because I'm a drug addict," I say. "I haven't done any drugs. I only do drugs recreationally a few times a year—on a quarterly basis at the most."

They laugh at me, repeating the words "*on a quarterly basis*" out loud. I laugh with them, but I know they don't believe me. I want to tell them to shut up, that I'm the face of someone who was abused and raped at the age of four. But I don't know that yet. So I stand there and let them snicker, believing what they want about me. I turn back around and wait to get the answer to my question. I can't have my medicine yet.

The other patients are all so nice to me. It seems like everyone in here wants to be my friend. An older, motherly-type woman in a brown sweater walks the halls with me. She comforts me. "I know they have a lot of rules here honey. But they have them for our protection. Learn what they are and how to follow them so you can get out of here sooner." I thank her for being so kind to me. She becomes my best friend in here for now. I tell her she is a gift from God to me because brown is my favorite color. Her brown sweater makes me feel relaxed. She smiles sweetly at me.

I start to try very hard to learn the rules. I stop pulling my shirt up and showing my boobs to people. I do my rituals and dances when they aren't looking. I gradually try to be quieter. I start doing what I'm told.

A case worker comes to see me. I tell her that I have a problem—that the staff people here keep telling me to go into my room and brush my hair when I've already done it. I tell her that it makes me angry to be told over and over to do something I've already done. "Alyssa, we can tell you are a pretty girl. And it looks like you don't care about yourself right now. It doesn't *look* like you've really brushed your hair. It still looks messy, and you walk around in the same clothes every day."

I tell her that I do care very much about myself. I tell her my body is in pain—that my brain is in pain. I am trying to survive. I tell her that I have naturally frizzy hair, but that I have indeed taken a shower and brushed it. I tell her that I have to wear the same clothes every day right now because they are what's comfortable, but that my family is taking them home every day for me and washing them for me. "I'm sorry I have frizzy hair, but I really don't have the energy to try and look like Angelina Jolie right now." I tell her that they are starting to hurt my feelings and make me feel self-conscious.

The case worker apologizes. "No one means to make you feel like you need to look like Angelina Jolie. But we do need to see that you care about your hygiene and appearance. How about you start putting your hair in a ponytail and putting on some lip gloss?"

I sit here stunned and deflated. She doesn't understand anything I just said. It's not enough for her that I said I took a shower, brushed my hair, and am wearing clean clothes. I need to *look* "put together"...as if without the proper female accessories I am not even fit to walk the halls of a United States mental hospital.

Thank God the medicines have started to balance my brain a little. Self control is something within my reach again. *Be quiet, Alyssa. Don't yell. Don't go on a rampage here. She's just doing her job. She's trying to meet you half way. Smile at her. Thank her for listening to you.* "Yes, I can do that," I politely agree.

What a fucked up world I live in. What ridiculous terms I am subject to. And people wonder why feminists can be so angry — calling us "raging" as if that is some sort of insult. I just looked into the eyes of a fellow human being, telling her that I am suffering in pain and fighting for my life, and she looked back and said, "Please wear a ponytail and lip gloss."

Maybe I *will* end up killing myself in here. I picture them coming to find my dead body in my room with a note that reads, "Here is your fucking ponytail." *No, it should be more subtle, Alyssa.* I'll write, "There, I did my hair." I laugh at the image in my mind. When you are fighting for your life, the sense of humor can get very dark. So I keep that joke to myself. And I ask my mom to please bring me hair accessories and lip gloss, and she does.

How can you subject me to this life, God? I don't know how I ended up here, but I know that domination and control are the forces behind it. I am losing my mind, my own sense of control, and everyone here tells me in order to get better I have to follow their rules. It feels like that same domination all over — like someone ran over me with a car and then put it in reverse and did it again.

Fuck this world you've created God! I hate everything about this life!!! Oh wait a minute...now I'm starting to get it, Jesus. Your body was broken too. You died by abuse for being yourself. You understand how I feel right now. You really do. Thank you. Please keep reminding me when I forget. I'll keep hanging on.

When my best friend here gets to go home before me, I am so happy for her. But I feel lonely too. God sends me a new friend, not someone who wears brown, but someone who is brown.

I stand in the day room staring at the TV, pretending that I am paying attention to it. "Hey," I hear a voice say. "Will you come over here and sit beside me for a minute?" I look over and see a large, tattooed man sitting on the couch and smiling at me.

"Sure." I walk over and sit beside him. "Can I ask you why you are in here?" he says to me. "Because I was raped," I blurt out. I don't even know if I just told him a lie or the truth, but the statement comes out before I can think about it. He nods and tells me that he understands. "How do you understand me?" I ask. "Were you in prison or something?" He says yes and tells me that he just got out. He asks me if I am afraid of him now. I say no. And I mean it.

He tells me that he thinks I'm beautiful, but that he doesn't mean it sexually. "There is something about you that makes me want to be your best friend," he tells me. "Will you be my best friend in here?" I say yes. He tells me that I'm smart…that he wants me to teach him everything I know, that he wants me to help him write a resume so he can get a job. He says, in turn, he will protect me and not let anything bad happen to me while we are in together. "You be the brains and I'll be the muscle," he says. I trust him.

My brown friend takes the time to observe me. He watches the way I pace the halls and perform my strange rituals. One day he tells me that he understands me and he joins me as I walk the hall. He performs my rituals with me. It makes me feel so good to be understood.

I begin to tune into him as well. He always has a smile and never admits to feeling anxiety. But I notice when the anxiety hits him and he breaks into a sweat. He needs me to walk with him sometimes and do rituals that comfort him. He asks me to walk four feet behind him so that he can feel my energy from a distance. When I walk behind him I notice that he walks very guarded with his hands crossed in protection over his ass. I know it is his prison walk and that he is protecting himself. I pray for him as I walk behind him, that he will feel healing and security.

I start to study the other patients too. We all learn each others' oddities and reach out to each other. The staff people here are nice, for the most part, but they don't *understand* insanity. The patients do. They keep me strong. In many ways I feel more love within these walls than I've ever felt anywhere else. It's weird how I can feel so fragile and scared, yet so loved at the same time.

My family comes to visit me every day for the full duration of visiting hours. I am so grateful. I can't survive without them. I notice I am the only one here with regular visitors. My fellow "inmates" notice too. My mom spends time with many of them because they don't have anybody. How do they survive? I admire them. They are the strong ones. Nothing about me feels strong right now. I need everything and everyone to help me survive.

Insanity, a Poem

Like a newborn, without cognition, relying only on her senses,
Will she be welcomed into the world with love and comfort?
Or will she be tossed aside, left to shiver in the cold, to die alone?
Insanity feels like the latter.
Everything I see is fuzzy. My senses turn on and off.
Sometimes the noises are too loud.
Sometimes I am deaf.
Everything tastes bitter or bland,
Yet I eat as fast as I can for fear that I'll starve.
No one makes sense to me, and I make sense to no one.
My confused adult mind is trapped inside my wounded body.
How do I find my way out of this maze?
No one understands my symbols, my code.
I must fight my own way out.
I talk in my head, talk to God and to my dead loved ones.
I pace the halls in certain patterns.
I create rituals and routines for myself.
So much anxiety runs through my veins,
I find no comfort in sitting, in laying down, in walking,
The effort to exist is excruciating.
I peer through the bars covering my window,

Aware that I'm a prisoner.
I haven't felt the sunlight or spring air in over a week.
The sane people are afraid I'll run away.
But I just want to be with my family.
When they come to visit,
I do happy dances in front of the glass as they sign in.
That way they can know I'm surviving.
I guess they don't understand my message though.
The case worker asks me how I feel about being in the hospital.
I'd rather be dead.
"When you answer that way honey,
they put you on suicide watch,
and you'll have to stay here longer," my family explains.
But, I didn't say I'm suicidal,
I said I'd rather be dead.
"Well, they don't see much difference,
so please stop saying that
if you want to get out of here," they coax.
I don't know what is wrong with me.
I only know I am in a maze of insanity
and I have to make it out. Today is the day that I do.
I still feel crazy as I sit here face to face with the woman who
holds the power to release me.
I know I have to play the game the right way.
This is the end of the rabbit hole.

One wrong answer
and I might be forced to spiral back through it.
"Call your family Alyssa, you can go home today."

Released

I can't believe I'm going home! Everything I see on the car ride home looks like something to be grateful for... the sunlight, the traffic lights, the strip malls...I feel like I have gotten lucky and somehow won a game of chess that my life depended on, without knowing any of the rules and strategies, or how I even wound up engaged in the game in the first place. My senses are overwhelmed with feelings of confusion, relief, and mental and physical exhaustion. I don't care right now that it will take me months, even years, to recover. This car ride home feels like the happiest moment of my life. I AM *FREE*.

Chapter Two: A Letter Unsent

"Forgiveness is the fragrance that the violet sheds on the heel that crushed it."

—*Mark Twain*

Dear Perpetrator,

I'm not ashamed that I've cried many tears over the fact that you have passed away, that I will never get the chance to see you again and ask you if you recognize my face.

I'm not ashamed to say that I loved you once. I was a four-year-old little girl. That was my nature, to give all the love and joy I had to everyone around me, including you.

I'm not ashamed to say I trusted you. Again, I was a four-year-old, and even all the grown-ups in our town trusted you. You worked hard establishing yourself in the community to gain that trust, holding positions of authority and respect. I thought you were someone powerful, and that I was your little buddy. I was so proud about that.

I'm not ashamed to say I feel sorry for you, because I know now that you were not strong at all. It is the weakest kind of man that must manipulate the innocent and command a little child to gratify him.

I'm not ashamed to say a small part of me almost thanks you for what you taught me. You taught me that the world can be brutal, that not everyone wants my smiles, my joy, and my love. Some people want to destroy me. Because of you, it wouldn't come as such a shock when that cold reality would shove me down again.

I'm not ashamed to say I hated you when I remembered. I wanted to get my revenge, nothing brutal, just sweet. I fantasized about meeting you at the scene of the crime and handcuffing you there, watching you feel the fear as I did. I imagined myself dressed provocatively, subjecting you to a grown up style lap dance, and feeling so elated when I felt the nothingness in your pants — because the woman I've become is someone too powerful for you to be attracted to. How I would have loved to clasp my hands gently around your throat, press my lips against your ear and whisper, "I'm taking your sunglasses off now, asshole. It's time to let the light shine in." Then I would have left you there.

And I'm not ashamed to say I've gotten to a place where I forgive you. That doesn't mean I absolve your actions. It doesn't mean I still love you. It doesn't mean that the anger will never return, or that I'll never feel the fear or the sorrow again. It simply means that I'm tired.

I've been tired my whole life...tired as a child from carrying your dirty secret...tired as a woman from the unleashing of it, so exhausted I couldn't even think about forgiving. And now I'm still tired, and probably always will be. But with every exhale, I let go of the grip you had over me. And with every inhale, I embrace that peace.

At first I couldn't believe that you were gone, though. How could you leave? How could you get away without being held accountable, without having to pay my medical bills, and without hearing my words? It felt like a cruel joke.

I wanted you to know everything about me, my accomplishments and my dreams. If I could just tell you how I survived all the pain you caused me, you would know that I'm stronger than you…and that I'm not just stronger than you now, but I was stronger than you when I was four years old.

But now I realize that you probably already knew that. And if you didn't, then there is nothing I could say to you now that could make you understand. And that's what other survivors have told me too…to just be grateful that you are gone, because I wouldn't get the response from you that I wanted if you were alive, or the justice.

So I'm left with only a fantasy of justice, the fantasy of sitting behind the microphone in a courtroom and saying these words to a jury:

"Thank you for hearing my case today. I am here because this man sexually abused and raped me. I have no traditional rape kit because it occurred over thirty years ago when I was a four-year-old girl, before I even knew what sex was.

Child abuse is a crime of convenience. It is to the perpetrator's benefit and advantage that memories many times take years to resurface, and that mental illness is often a result. The defense can claim that the very repercussions of this man's actions in my life are what make my testimony unreliable. So I offer you my evidence in hopes that you will trust it upon review.

I submit to you my medical records. You can read the details of the mental anguish this man has caused me. I submit to you statements from my counselor about how the knowledge came about over the course of our sessions. You can ask me about the nightmares and the flashbacks. You can touch my body, hold my hands and feel them tremble from the fear that is trapped in my body all these years later.

My body is the rape kit. My life is the rape kit."

And the fantasy of addressing you directly from behind that same microphone:

"All these years, you thought I was obediently complying with your command of silence. But I was simply waiting for the right moment to speak.

I almost died because of you....from the sheer terror of you. I've wanted to end my life at times because of the pain that's housed in my body. You almost took my sanity for good. They told my family there was a 50% chance I might have to be locked away forever.

But I'm here. And you didn't stop me from living, from laughing, or from loving.

Do you remember looking into my young eyes and telling me it was just like sucking a thumb? I became an animal in that moment, as I smelled the deception in your loins.

What you did to me could have destroyed any ability in me to open my heart up to a man, but it didn't. You could have destroyed my ability to trust a man with my body, but you didn't. You acted by manipulation, coercion, force, and threats over my life. Maybe you only knew monsters in your own life. Maybe you were never shown what a man looked like and acted like. So, I'd like to tell you about mine.

He is a man who considers me his best friend, first and foremost. A man who respected the innocent things about me, not wanting to destroy that innocence as you did. He is a man who stands up for me and would have stood up to you on my behalf. He is a man who defended me over the years, when people said I was weird or called me names like "slut" and "tease." He is a man who has stood by me through the past several years of turmoil you have caused me...a man who has never uttered a bad word about me to anyone, even at times when it could be warranted...a man who has endured the repercussions of your influence in our marriage with grace and strength...a man, who though exhausted, has stood by me as I've struggled to figure myself out, and let me be myself without judgment...a man who understands what forgiveness is...a man who never throws my mistakes in my face, or repays evil with evil. A man with a gentle, compassionate nature whose heart aches over all the sorrows in the world...a man who loves me enough to commit himself to me, so that we can negotiate life in this crazy world together.

He is my best friend, and a protection. I love to act silly and try to make him laugh. I love to take walks with him and our dog. I love to feel his presence beside me in the bed. I love to put my head on his chest and feel him breathing. I like the rare times he obliges me by scratching my back with his face stubble or when he scratches my arms for me. I like the fact that he waters our flowers and walks in the yard giving loving attention to our trees that we planted. I like how he heats up our dog's food on the stove for him in the mornings. How he cooks breakfast for me before I go to work on a Saturday. How he cares for me when I'm sick. I like how he searches for movies and puts them in the cue so that we always have a full selection of something interesting to watch. I like how he sends me articles to read, and helps me stay up to date on things going on in the world. I like that he enjoys life's simple pleasures with me.

He is my man. I trust him with my love, with my body, and with my life. He is not perfect, and he does not have to be. There is not one thing about him that could ever be anything like you.

I wish you could have known love like that in your life, because then maybe you wouldn't be sitting here now. Maybe all the good things that everyone in the community felt about you would really be true."

But I'll never get to say those words. And you'll never read this letter. Or the following poem that I wrote before I forgave you:

"The Sickness of You"

Snatched, sucked down into the pit
Like quick sand, the feces that is your soul engulfed me
Suffocating me, feces pouring into my ears, my nostrils,
Getting underneath my eyelids,
Filling my mouth,
Even entering my lungs as I inhaled
I prayed not to die
Knowing if I inhaled one more time that I would
Please God, lift me up from this Pit
My prayer was heard
I was lifted up
I opened my eyes and could see the light
Gasping for breath I cried out

Where is the holy water?

I need to be cleansed

I washed you off, but a part of you settled inside me

The feces that filled my mouth found its way to my colon

It settled there and hardened like plaque

Over the years it has slowly been seeping,

Permeating every cell in my body

I am contaminated

I need to purge

There is a shit deep inside me that is you

When I allow myself to feel the fear of you, I have to shit

Now I'm learning that I can let go of that fear

But how do I get you out of me?

I can't shit enough times to rid myself of you

When people ask me how I really feel, I say

I feel like I need to vomit,

And when I do, I'm going to spew feces from my mouth.

I don't feel that way anymore. Through forgiveness, I've purged. My spirit is clean, and I am working on being the person that I want to be. But the shit of you has impacted me forever. My nervous system and brain chemistry are permanently changed. That used to piss me off. But now I just tell myself, "When life hands you shit, fertilize a garden."

Chapter Three: The Puzzle of a Shattered Psyche

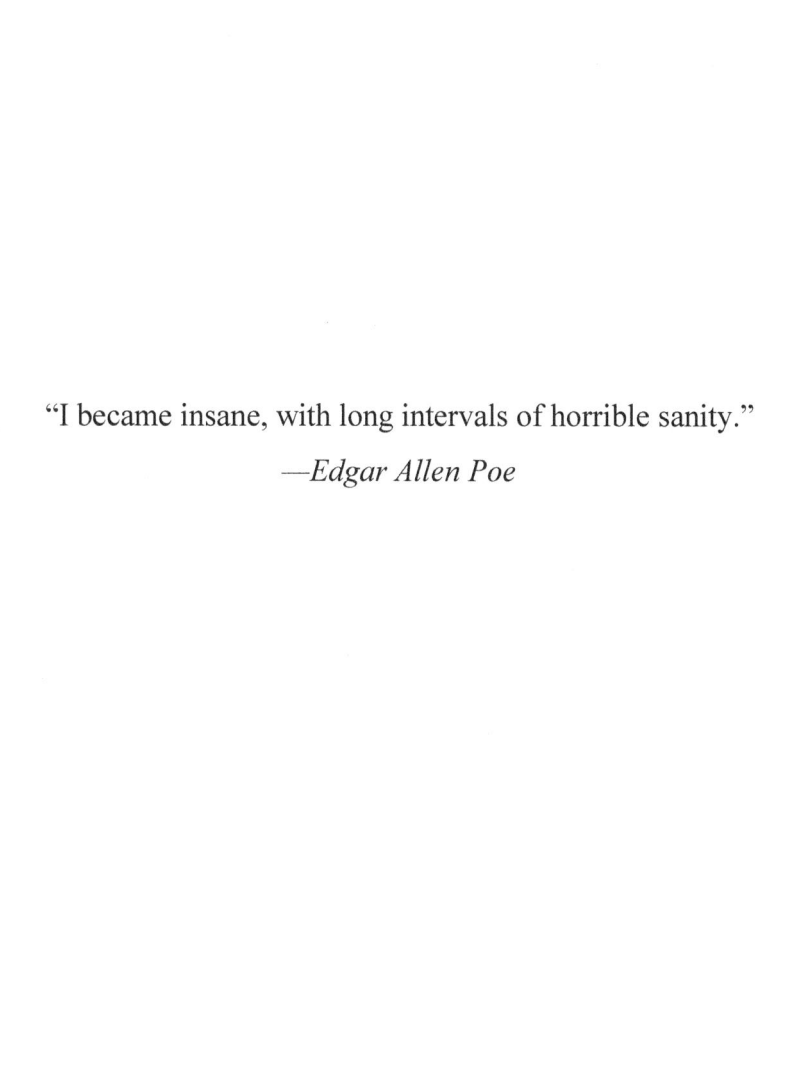

"I became insane, with long intervals of horrible sanity."
—*Edgar Allen Poe*

On the Counselor's Couch

Sanity can be its own kind of torture. It leaves us with the daunting task of making sense of the madness—facing what sent us to the hell of insanity in the first place.

Being in the hospital left me with having to practice how to do basic things from scratch again. Everything required effort: Reading, writing, household chores, grocery shopping, driving, and eventually going back to work.

My body and my brain still hurt, but the sleep that I had lacked felt so good…like when I closed my eyes all fear was melting away and every cell in my body was turning over with restoration.

As directed by the hospital, I kept up with my continued care appointments and stayed on the medication plan. At times, though, sadness overwhelmed me. I would cry to my husband, apologizing for being such a drain on him and for being so useless. He would never say much, just hug me, and tell me that I would get better.

My counselor explained that what happened to me is sort of like a computer crashing. All the files in my brain had gotten mixed up. Recent memories could be mixed up with childhood memories, and so on. "I'm going to help you sort through the files and re-organize everything, Alyssa. We're going to work very carefully and slowly, so that you don't have any flashbacks and wind up back in the hospital. Don't be scared of this process. You have experienced some traumas in life, but your brain has protection mechanisms so you don't have to remember anything you aren't ready for or don't ever want to remember. But you strike me as a person who isn't going to stop until you get everything figured out." I nodded my head in agreement, but I told him that I wasn't completely sure. "I might be too scared to remember everything."

Our first sessions focused on the hospitalization and preceding events: When I started feeling like something was wrong with me, when the depression and manic signs started. We sorted through the pieces of traumas that had started coming out during the hospitalization. He explained that things I remembered in a depressive state may have been more traumatic in actuality than I remembered, and that things I recalled while in a manic state may be over-exaggerated in my brain. And so we began the process of sorting all that out.

I have been so grateful for his help, for someone willing to listen to me and help me with my process. He helps me dissect my past, make peace with my present, and find hope for my future.

Through our sessions, I've begun to face...

My Fears

I fear being asked questions. When someone asks me more than two questions in a row, I feel like I am standing in front of a firing squad — each question a deadly bullet. I can't even think of the answer; I only think about deflecting the informational assault. I fear being commanded or told what to do in general. I fear my compliance makes me subject to mind control. Likewise, I fear asking for what I want and getting it, like it's some sort of power I don't want to possess. I fear if we humans aren't careful, we can be shut down, becoming robots, even when the intent might be loving.

I fear being forgotten, but I fear how people might remember me. I fear being noticed and I fear being invisible. I fear eyes moving over my body. I fear being attractive and I fear being unattractive. I fear existence and I fear ceasing to exist. I fear everything about myself.

I feel like my physical body is just a host for some foreign being residing in it…like I have no idea who I am or what reality is anymore. What if what my counselor calls "protection mechanisms" is really my mind playing tricks on me? What if everything I know to be true has been a lie? This scares me, to no longer feel like I can trust my own grasp of reality. I have to tune into other people's gauges. I have to fit myself into check boxes that psychiatrists have designed to determine what "normal range" for mood and behavior is.

My counselor has me do homework between sessions—breathing, mindfulness, and writing exercises. He teaches me coping skills for stress and my fears. Some of what I do exceeds his expectations and he doesn't hold back in telling me that. "Alyssa, you are a joy to work with. People don't come into my office talking about the kind of trauma and afflictions you have faced with such astuteness and with brightness on their faces like you have." When I tell him I feel like a failure to my husband, my employer, my family, and friends, he tells me that I am attractive intellectually, physically, and spiritually. Even on days when I feel close to suicidal, like hurting myself, or wishing I would get hit by a bus, he just smiles, like he has faith in me, and tells me to make an appointment to come back and see him soon.

Most of the time, his words uplift me. He gives me hope, and I enjoy going to him so much more than to my medication management appointments at the shrink's office. But some days I really wonder, what is this brightness on my face people see when they look at me? Where does it come from? Would I have to actually kill myself for people to finally grasp how sad I really am on the inside? Would I have to stay permanently institutionalized for people to comprehend how much fear resides in my body? A cute smile can be a curse. The body we are housed in doesn't protect us from the plague of invisibility.

I never have bad thoughts about my counselor though. He is compassionate and dedicates his time to help people like me through difficult life processes. But some days going to see him depresses me. I contemplate our modernized culture. I think about superficiality and greed. It feels like no one wants to listen to pain. We glorify it, sure, on the news, but we don't *listen* to it and we don't *advocate* en mass for the broken. We brush everything under the rug, pretending that life can be okay for all of us if we as individuals just have enough self-determination. We live in a culture where everything is bought and sold, even compassion. And for the ones who can't afford it, it often isn't there for them.

But I stick with the therapy program because I'm fortunate enough to have one. And despite my various soap boxes, it is helping me.

Hiding Inside My Mind with Phantom

My counselor and I talk more about this feeling I have that I am not at home inside my own body. That I feel like a guest in my own house, and that when I am in certain social situations, I feel like I am not directly there, but rather an observer, watching the conversations and events unfold like a movie.

"Someone hurt you very badly when you were young, Alyssa. What you are describing is called an out-of-body experience. They can be quite common for victims of childhood trauma," he explains. He is careful not to feed me misguided information, but he asks me pointed questions about that sensation and about my past. He asks me questions about my childhood. Can I remember smells, tastes, or colors pertaining to childhood experiences?

At first, I can't remember much of anything. I tell him my childhood is pretty blurry. But over time, little pieces keep coming to the surface, like pieces of a puzzle. For a long time, I just collect all the pieces and look at them, think about them, and write about them. I try to arrange them and can never get the image quite right. I know something traumatic and abusive happened, but I don't know the "what" or the "who." So we begin to talk about what I remember.

I talk about the loneliness I felt as a little girl, how in preschool the other girls wouldn't let me play with them. My only friend was the boy who sat beside me. He would invite me to play outside with the other boys, but I would just stand under a tree by myself and watch them run around wrestling. I was grateful though that he at least cared about me and wanted to be my friend.

That became a comfortable trend for me, becoming a mere observer of other's socialization and only getting close to one person at a time that I could trust and feel close to. It was around that time that I met my ghost. I call her my Phantom. She was born out of fear and came to life when I was four years old. She holds the full memory of the abuse that happened to me.

The first time I remember meeting her, I was running to my mom for comfort because I was scared of going to sleep. I realized that I had jumped out of my body and was watching myself run down the hall. Once I realized I could do that, it became a game I would play with myself, jumping outside of myself when I ran down the stairs. Phantom and I would race each other, but she would always jump back inside my body once I reached the bottom step so we would end in a tie.

In my elementary years, Phantom and I didn't play that game anymore. She was content to sit inside my body, focusing her attention on other misfits like myself—the girl who frequently peed her pants in class, the boy who sat across from me with no friends that people teased because they said he smelled, and the girl who sat in front of me who had raw, scaly patches on her scalp.

I never joined in the laughter or teasing. I just sat and quietly watched, soaking every scene in like a sponge. It was as if Phantom was trying to tap me on the shoulder and get my attention, nudging me to take note of what I had in common with these lonely souls.

As I watched that boy walk to his house when he got off the bus at his stop, I imagined being his friend and seeing what life was like inside his house. And I envied the girl in my class with the scaly scalp. I wanted to have an open wound that I could pick at, something others considered unsightly. And as I observed the puddle of urine forming under the other girl's seat during class, I felt sorry for her.

Phantom was reminding me about the time I had shit myself at home. I was too old for that, so I hid it from my parents…throwing away my underwear, wiping myself with my doll blanket, and keeping it in the doll crib my dad had built for me. Every once in a while I would check on it. Check to see when it had dried out. Check to see when it stopped smelling. Check to see when the brown faded and it became less noticeable over time.

Phantom tried to speak for me a few times. She tried to get her message out, but no one understood.

I sat at the dinner table staring at the hot dog I was given for dinner. I couldn't eat it. Something about it looked wrong. It reminded me of something, but I didn't know what. I couldn't stand the sight of it, the texture of it, and putting it in my mouth made me feel physically sick. So I hid it in my pants and sat quietly in my bedroom waiting for my dad to come and kill me. I was always thinking I might make a man angry enough to kill me. Phantom was trying to tell my parents that.

"How is the little blind boy in Alyssa's Sunday school class?" my grandma asked my mom. "I've been praying for him every night."

"What? What are you talking about? There's no blind boy in Alyssa's class."

"Are you sure? She told me all about it when she spent the night here. She said she's the only one who will be his friend and that she helps him cross the street."

Phantom had told a lie, except the truth was wrapped up inside. Phantom was trying to tell the grown-ups that I was blind, but she was helping me. She was asking them to notice and to help. But they didn't know what she was talking about anymore than I did.

Phantom stood up for me too. She fought back.

A boy in my class had his eye on me and made it clear that he wanted to beat me up. It was probably just a case of first-grade love. Funny, how even at such a young age, love and pain are so intertwined. I remember the smile he used to flash at me as he walked by my desk. He knew I was safe there and so did I. But during recess, he had the power to torment. And to his pleasure, I ran. I ran until I couldn't stand it anymore. And that was the day Phantom helped me.

He and I stood face to face. All the kids had gathered around to see the fight. "Okay, if you want to punch me, go ahead." And he did, directly in the gut. I stumbled backwards as the wind was knocked out of me. Fury flooded my body. The anger at the pain he inflicted kept me from crying. The punch I threw back, much to my surprise, hit him square in his face. I stood wide-eyed as I watched his top lip swell up and start to bleed. How had I just done that? As the kids shouted and cheered, my first-grade enemy burst into tears in front of everyone. From that day forward, I could play in peace. I had faced my fear and I had won.

It's funny, when you feel so alone inside, the whole world can love you but you don't know it.

I got invited to birthday parties and other girls' houses for sleepovers, but I felt so lonely that I had no idea I was invited because people actually liked me. I thought maybe they were inviting me to make fun of me or because their parents forced them to. I was always very reserved and quiet, pretty much just waiting for the shindig to be over so I could go home.

In sixth grade, I found out what it felt like to have zero friends instead of one or two. We had moved to a new town 1,000 miles away from where I'd grown up. Being teased for being different…standing completely alone on a playground during recess and just wishing I could fast forward time until the end of the day when I could go home—this was now my reality. One really is the loneliest number.

Over time though, being 1,000 miles away from where the abuse had happened gave Phantom the ability to go further into hiding, giving my physical self room to flourish. I formed meaningful friendships and had typical teenage fun, truly *feeling* happy. The signs were still there: the avoidance of boys, the dark poetry I'd write, an occasional hallucination or nightmare, the sleeping 12 hours a day…but I smiled, laughed, and sang and danced so much that no one noticed.

Phantom would not show herself again until I had my breakdown. I had only played with her as a child. We had never had a conversation before. But it was in my time of madness that she spoke as she hovered above my body. She was so powerful; I felt that the strength of her pull could cause me to die. "Why are you trying to kill me?" I asked her. "I'm not trying to kill you, Alyssa. I'm trying to protect you from this. You can't handle it. You can trust me. It's okay to just let go and come with me into the light."

I lay there in my bed, looking up at her and then over at my husband. Could I trust her? Could I really die right now and go to heaven?

"I believe you, but I can't go with you now. I have to hold on. If I go with you now, my husband won't know why I died. I can't watch him go through that grief. If I can't survive this, I will at least hang on long enough for him to know what killed me. I need you to leave me alone now." And she did.

Moment of Awareness

After talking through the memories with my counselor, I still don't believe I'll ever be able to remember the full truth about whatever abuse occurred, and I tell my counselor that. *How* can I? *How* will the memories come back? "Just keep relaxing, don't stress about it, and you'll eventually remember what you need to," he tells me. And he's right. The day comes that I do remember.

In that moment of awareness, my body goes into convulsions. I call him and tell him I need to come see him as soon as possible. Thankfully, he has an open appointment for me. I drive there in a panic. I keep making wrong turns. All around me there seem to be signs of what happened to me when I was four years old. *I have to make it there*, I think. *Don't run off the road. Just breathe, drive, and get there.*

I burst into his office, still trembling. I tell him what I remembered and how difficult the drive to his office was for me. I tell him that if this memory had come back a year ago, I would have ended up back in the hospital. I would not have been able to drive to his office.

At my words he hugs me, then takes both of my hands and we sit down face to face. He bursts into tears. "I am so proud of you and happy for you, Alyssa. I know it's painful right now, but you are making so much progress." His sincerity, and the fact that a grown man would unashamedly cry tears of sorrow and joy over me, is one of the most beautiful moments I have in my memory bank.

Mental Illness and Me

I used to be known as a sweet, quiet girl with a kind smile. The few people who got close to me would see my silly side sometimes, or even get a glimpse of the caged wild woman longing to break free. Now everyone who knows me has just about seen it all. That was a large part of my mental crisis. The breakdown represented more than a chemical imbalance and memories of abuse that were surfacing.

I was a fractured person and didn't even know it. Because of the secret I had carried since childhood, I thought I had to hide everything about myself. I thought the very people I cared most about would cease to love me if they knew who I really was. Consequently, I continued the painful habit of keeping secrets.

Keeping secrets is a burden, and when I finally ended up in the hospital because of it, I lost the ability to hide anything about myself. In my mania, I prattled on to my conservative Christian parents about my past drug use. I bossed my agnostic husband around, instructing him to research Bible verses for me and study their meaning. And I showed my naked body unashamedly to people. I was loud and dramatically comical, depressed, angry, perverse, spiritual, sexually overt, a fearless woman, yet a completely wounded and terrified child all at once.

Everything happened like a tornado, and I'm still dealing with the aftermath. And it feels like even when there's a long period of calm in my life, I still always feel that the climate is right within me for another storm to rage.

They say that's what I need medicine for now. That's what I need counseling for. That's what I need regimented routine, exercise, and healthy habits for. I need to keep mood journals, log my feelings, my sexual appetite, my behavior patterns and sleep patterns…anything and everything to keep another tornado from wreaking havoc in my life, destroying myself and the people I care about.

It took me a long time to make peace with the fact that I am now a person with labels—labels that scare people. I didn't want to believe what all the psychiatrists said…that my diagnosis is serious, even dangerous.

I didn't feel like a person when I would sit down on the psychiatrist's couch and have to answer questions like: "On a scale of 1 to 10, how depressed are you?" "Have you cheated on your husband?" "Do you hallucinate or hear voices that aren't really there?" "Do you have a gun in your house?" "Do you have thoughts of harming yourself or others?"

And I didn't feel human when they told me the medication choices: "This medicine may make you gain 40 pounds in a month's time, or this one may make your hair fall out; that one may give you permanent muscle twitches, and it can make men grow breasts."

I just sat there in quiet frustration, thinking, "These are the options that are supposed to help people with low self-esteem who are already on a dangerous mental ledge feel better and live healthier lives?"

But over time, I came to realize that the doctors were just doing their jobs. And that job is to deliver the cold hard facts. They tell you the diagnosis, the dangers, the treatments paths, and the risks. And for things like hope and encouragement, they refer out.

Once I started making peace with how our system works, I could begin to appreciate and even embrace the information the doctors were delivering to me. And the facts are that I have two mental illnesses that cannot be cured. Some people do recover from PTSD, but since I have had it since age four, my brain chemistry has been altered for so long that the damage is permanent. And Bipolar 1 Disorder also is something I will have to live with forever.

The medicines can manage the symptoms, but even with medication there are risks: Side effects, or the body can build up tolerances, or they may cause episodes of the very conditions they are trying to control, like mania and depression. The facts are that there is always a risk I could end up in the hospital again, become suicidal again.

The facts are that, statistically, my marriage has a 90% chance of failure.

Even when I began embracing the facts, it still took me a while to get over the delusion that I could conquer these diseases if I just had enough will power. So against my doctor's recommendations, I tried just that. I quit taking my medicine. I thought if I could heal emotionally from the trauma and make peace with my life, I wouldn't need to take the medicine anymore. I thought my brain would intuitively know that there was no need for me to hallucinate, now that it had unleashed the reason for why I went crazy in the first place. I honestly felt like knowing the truth about myself and making peace with it would mean I was no longer mentally ill.

But, just like the doctor predicted, my experiment failed. I had another manic episode. Fortunately, I am not too proud to admit when I'm wrong. On the third day of not sleeping, when I felt my brain spiraling in uncontrollable circles, I called my doctors and immediately started back on the medicine. I had to take a week off from work to stabilize, but I didn't end up back in the hospital. It scared me enough though to bring me to a place of full acceptance…that I am a person who needs to take medicine for the rest of my life.

When I went to see my counselor, I told him about the experience. He said, "Alyssa, there is nothing wrong with taking medicine. Because of the trauma that happened to you, you are a person who just needs to wear a brace on your brain, that's all." I liked the way that sounded and the imagery. So that's how I choose to view it now.

But having an invisible brace on my brain for an invisible disability can make life challenging sometimes. It means sometimes people will think I'm stupid when I get overwhelmed by the simplest question or when I can't understand an instruction or see a sign that's right in front of me. So I have to either become okay with being viewed as stupid sometimes or become comfortable expressing the fact that I have an invisible disability.

Having an invisible disability means my husband will experience frustration sometimes when he's ready to get a jumpstart on the day and I need to take several hours to get over the nightmares I woke up from. It means that strangers will think I'm weird when I cry in public for no apparent reason. It means sometimes people might think I'm being lazy when I just need extra time to rest. And it means that I will never be able to "get over it" because no matter how much emotional peace I achieve, the trauma will continue to be replayed in my brain and body over and over again.

But cold hard facts don't have to mean life is hopeless. I can choose to live a healthy life to the best of my ability. I can nurture my sanity with my medications. I can exercise and feed my body healthy foods. I can fight to be in the 10% category of marriages that make it. With every day that I'm afforded, I can live with determination. I can choose laughter and love.

So what is Rape Anyways?

Rape: "Penetration, no matter how slight, of the vagina or anus with any body part or object, or oral penetration by a sex organ of another person, without the consent of the victim."

According to the above definition from the "Rape, Abuse, and Incest National Network," I have been raped three times in my life – twice orally and once anally – twice with a threat of murder over my life.

It's taken me so many years to come to terms with that reality because most people in our culture still don't seem to understand the definition. Likewise, our legal systems are not designed to execute law in full support of the definition. Definitions and penalties vary from state to state. Time and time again, victims who choose to report are turned away and told any number of absurd things by professionals who either do not understand the definition themselves, or do understand but choose not to care.

So consequently, for many years I really had no idea I was raped. After all, his dick never went *all the way in* to my asshole, right? By some miracle, I was able to deflect a painful assault by continuing to make out with him and sweet talk my way out of the situation. He fell asleep. I made my escape, and no substantial physical pain occurred. Never mind that I had been backed against a wall, cornered, told I was not permitted to leave, and that it was either have sex with him or he would murder me right then with his bare hands. And never mind that I left trembling, running for my life into the blackness of the night.

And again with the oral assault, I thought because there was no physical pain, I wasn't really raped. At worst, he was just a douchebag and things like that happen at parties. I was drunk, said yes to going into the bedroom, and should have been smarter. At best, maybe he was just initiating some sort of rough sexual play. Maybe if I hadn't been such a sheltered Christian girl, had more education and experience, I might have been able to handle myself better and perhaps even enjoyed it...???

At the time, I didn't realize that I actually did have past sexual experience—that I had been orally raped and threatened with murder at the age of four, and that history was simply repeating itself.

Who I See in the Mirror

I don't always see myself as an abuse survivor or identify as a rape victim. I think because my memories surfaced in recent adulthood, the knowledge that had been buried caused me to relate to all kinds of people who've experienced similarly isolating pain.

When I look in the mirror, I see the old woman lying in her refuse and waiting for the nurses' aide to come. I see the abandoned street child. I see the prisoner all alone in his cell of solitary confinement. I see the villager who felt the earth's tremble from the drone strike. I see the homeless man who struggles with his mental illness and can't get his medical needs met. I see the runaway teenager. I see the kidnapped and the tortured. I see the hermaphrodite and the eunuch. I see the untouchables, the invisible, and the forgotten. When people look into my blue eyes, I want them to know who is really looking back.

There was a day I looked in the mirror and saw my childhood abuser staring back at me, clear as day. I clenched my hands on my bathroom sink, put my face up to the mirror, and with a rage that rose from my gut said, "Fuck You!" right to his face. That felt so good.

But I've pondered that moment and wondered, why did I see his image in my own reflection? Had his demons become mine? Is there a perpetrator in all of us? I thought about the times I've been deceptive, manipulative, a thief, a liar, and a cheat. There is a bit of a perpetrator in me that I had to acknowledge, but I am not an abuser. I am striving to change my negative habits, and to bring my darkness to the light. And with every day I will keep reinventing myself until I like who I am.

Laughing at My Life

I spend an immeasurable amount of time in my life trying to reconcile the darkness of existence. And I always come back to the two things that help me continue to survive it: Having an active imagination and taking a step back to find something to laugh at every day. I'm convinced that my guardian angel is a grumpy old man who chain smokes. For the most part, he does a kick-ass job of protecting me in life and he can effectively smoke and work at the same time. But everyone needs to sit down and take a break from time to time…so I don't hold it against my guardian angel for needing to look the other way every now and again.

Of course, I know there are much more sophisticated ways of answering the age old questions like "What is the meaning of life?" and "Why do bad things happen to good people?" But, imagining a heaven full of angels who chain smoke, works for me. It's how I put the senselessness of life into a laughable context.

I even go so far as to imagine myself entering the pearly gates upon my death and bumping into my childhood abuser. In the scene I smile, punch him in the arm, and say, "Rape me now, motherfucker." And we both share a good laugh. It's hardly Biblical, or scientific. But, it's my very own comical afterlife fantasy.

Being silly and comical was something I had to learn. I grew up around moody men—whether it be just the gloomy demeanors that accompany generalized depression, or whether it be a full-scale alcoholic rage. It was the women in my family who taught me how to laugh at life and how to persevere. My mom is a bundle of sweetness...a soft place to fall for everyone in our family. She is always ready to soothe and bring comfort to a situation. But, she is also the one who taught me to delicately "tip-toe" around a man's moods, a habit that I am still un-learning.

It was my two closest aunts who I also looked up to as shining examples of the depth of strength that a female can embody. They are no strangers to life experiences like sexual assault, abandonment, domestic violence, addictions, divorce, and loss. But through the darkness of life, their spirits shine.

My mom's sister is sixty. She used to be a disco-queen and she still dresses up for Halloween every year. She is always ready to tell a funny story and eagerly anticipates the moment when everyone in the room bursts into laughter, including herself. She is the woman who taught me what real sex appeal is. She has style, fashion sense, and a magnetic personality. Ever since I was young, I hoped I could be as sexy as her someday.

My dad's sister is equally sexy and fierce, but with a different quality about her. When I was a little kid, she was my buddy. I couldn't wait for her to come to visit and take me out for Chinese food and bowling. We'd go as a family to the amusement park and she would be the one to never tire of riding all the fast rides with me. She is tough, and really knows how to throw a baseball and football, not just "push the ball into the air" as I tend to do. All my life she tried to teach me how, but I've never mastered it. She's over 60 now, and is still in phenomenal shape. She could outrun me any time. If I was ever in danger, she is the woman I would want by my side. I always knew she was a fighter, and that she would fight for me like a mother bear if I ever needed her to.

Through years of watching the women I love laugh their way through life, I learned the art form too. I laugh at my own mental illness many times. I laugh when I get so shaky that I spill food all over myself. I laugh when my PTSD flare-ups cause my senses to go into overdrive. I can smell foul things miles away, once even smelling my husband's fart *before* he farted.

I live on a time delay, so I laugh when I answer a question five minutes after the fact and the person forgets what they even asked me. I laugh at my own neurosis and paranoia. I laugh during the full moon when I have to put myself on house arrest so that I won't go on a horny bipolar rampage and hump everyone in the whole town.

Every comedian likes to have an audience. And for the most part, I like mine to be small. I feel satisfied when I crack an unexpected joke and make my co-workers laugh or make my husband smirk after he's had a bad day. But there are days when I want the whole world to be my stage and to hear my story.

I guess maybe some people who've never had to keep such a dark secret bottled up can't fully understand the need I have for self-exposure. I was trying to explain it to my brother…how I felt like people weren't real and everyone was superficial. He said, "Alyssa, you have to have filters for parts of yourself. You can't show your true self to everyone all the time because people at the grocery store don't care that you're bipolar. As a whole, people *are* caring, and that's why there are support groups you can go to where you can talk about those kinds of things."

And I can understand his point. It's not like it would be fair to people to bombard everyone with my whole life story. And I don't want to do that. But I do have certain random urges to be real. Like at the grocery store when the clerk is ringing up my produce and asks me how I'm doing, sometimes I'd like to reply, "Well, getting raped sucks, but thank God I can still laugh at a cucumber."

A Church Girl With X-Rated Material

A church girl with X-rated material. That's what I like to call myself. It describes my experience in a way that makes me smile. Viewing my life as a dark comedy helps me let go of the resentment that I have carried with me for so long. I've felt like my power of sexual choice was hijacked, first by my childhood abuser, and second by religious indoctrination which reinforced the notion that sexuality is something to be controlled.

Though I hated aspects of religious control, God has always been a natural and easy concept for me to embrace...I guess because of the fact that a human did such a terrible thing to me when I was so young. Even though my vocabulary wasn't developed yet, from the time I could think, I was aware that humans didn't have all the answers...that we are fallible beings who disappoint, that we live in a world where good and evil become intertwined and distorted. I wanted to believe in something that was eternally dependable, eternally loving, and a God that would never change his mood towards me.

Because of that sincere desire, I carved out my own relationship with God from the time I was very young. Even though I was a "good little girl" who always did as I was told, it was in my own mind where I felt the freedom to defy. Because of the abuse, I grew up thinking I had no choice but to obey authority. But from the time I could form my own thoughts, I knew that's what they were…MINE. And even God himself couldn't force me to blindly believe in him. So, I challenged God directly in a sweet four-year-old way, threatening him with my prayers, "God if you don't send me an angel, I will never believe in you." And though modern science may very well label it an early childhood bipolar hallucination, an angel paid me a visit to my room one night. And since that day, I have believed.

It's hard to fit into a societal box though, to feel accepted, when you're a church girl with X-rated material. It's difficult to sit in church listening to sermons about sexual purity and saving yourself for marriage when you've already had sex at the age of four. And it's difficult to listen to the judgment that often comes from the pulpit about the lifestyles of everyone presumed to be going to hell. Even though my memories of abuse were repressed during the years I grew up in church, my questioning nature was strengthening as a result.

Church seemed to promote the same message I had received as a little girl: Sexuality needs to be shrouded in secrecy, and obey the rules or be punished. It became obvious to me over time that though church was full of sincere, well-intentioned people, it was a house of secrets and a house of judgment. I just wanted it to be a house of love.

I kept waiting for that sermon. How can love really transform people? What does it look like when love is played out in our lives? Can love truly liberate us? How do we fight for justice and lift up the oppressed? Sometimes my questions were touched on. But most often, God seemed to be portrayed as some Santa Claus in the sky who is checking our list to see if we have been naughty or nice.

It is easier to judge than to acknowledge. It is easier to preach than to educate. So week after week we sat in church, hiding our own humanity. Hiding the abuse within our walls, the disintegrating sanctity of our own marriages, the depression, the addictions, the gluttony, the greed, and the pride. We raised our hands and danced, saying our reverent prayers, and pretending we had a message of hope for the world.

Disappointingly, God also sounded a lot like an abuser to me: Someone who says he loves you, but then gets angry and punishes you for not obeying, then says he loves you again, sends you a gift with supposedly no strings attached, but then if you are leery of it or don't accept it in time, he gets angry again and painfully punishes you for all eternity.

I was a church girl with X-rated material and so many questions.

But when I ran from church, I only found a world just as eager to smack me down. A world that many times made me feel like my faith was silly or naïve. And a world that was waiting to manipulate and abuse. I was ill-prepared to face that reality. And I was devastated. I had taken the concept of love that I cherished from my spiritual upbringing and run to the world looking for practical answers to my questions. In my exuberance to live in freedom and enjoy the world as a playground, I only found myself crushed and confused all over again. Consequently, seeds of bitterness grew within me. But as I'm maturing and making peace with the past, I realize that it's never too late to write my own definitions.

So I have defined my God as "Infinite Love." My God has big shoulders. He doesn't need me to stroke his ego. He doesn't need me to agree with him, or think or behave in a certain way to reinforce who he is. My God is strong. He can handle my bad language and laugh at my dirty jokes. He was there after all when I prayed in those darkest moments of sexual assault. The creator of the universe has it under control. Infinite Love never has mood swings.

I have defined my life as a dark comedy. I find it all tragically hilarious.

I define myself as a church girl with X-rated material. And I define my liberation as exposing my darkness to those who are blinded by the light while continuing to shine brightly on those in this world who desire to snuff it out.

A Strange Kind of Healing

Just because I say I'm putting things behind me for good, and this book is helping me to do so, doesn't mean "I'm all better now." It doesn't mean I'll never shed another tear over my past. It doesn't mean I'll always be the perfect wife. I've never thought in linear terms. I view things in circles. It's not like I can put trauma, breakdown, healing, and whole person on a straight line. Things happen all at once sometimes. There is love happening in the midst of trauma. There is growth happening in the face of immaturity. And I'm sure even when I'm an old lady, there will be times when I cry over the four-year-old little girl inside me.

My counselor told me something that has been very helpful. He said, "Alyssa, being healed doesn't always mean living without medicine, or the absence of symptoms. You may have certain manifestations of what happened that stay with you for your whole life and you might not. But it's how you choose to conduct yourself in the midst of that, and how you choose to live your life in spite of it all that matters. When you choose to pursue a happy, healthy life you are living with the mindset of healing."

I will carry those words with me always. Having battle wounds that are still throbbing keeps me connected to people that are in the midst of the fight. It keeps my empathy and my compassion flowing at full force. I'm a veteran of some violent battles, and I will always carry in my heart my fellow warriors who are still fighting through the abuse. To every infant, toddler, child, teenager, woman and man who is surviving, I applaud you.

"Through all the tears
And all the fears
We often times may hear
The crunching sound of broken glass
Beneath the feet of God
As he walks about
Treading upon the broken hearts
Of his people;
The pieces, he says, to be cast as stars
Across the canopy of a night time sky."

A Poem Written by my Dad, 1996

Epilogue

I glance over at my husband as we sit side by side in the car. This time, I don't feel fear when I look at him. I'm filled with gratitude that I've made it this far—that I'm well enough to go on another road trip, and that I have a friend who has stood by me.

I sit quietly and contemplate the past couple of years—all the anguish, and all the hard work of putting the shattered pieces of myself back together. It all seems surreal. I think about the terror of it all.

"If I ever go that crazy again, I'm gonna need you to mix up a suicide cocktail, drive me to the beach, lay me down in the sand, and hold me as I drink it so I can die peacefully in the sun listening to the sound of the ocean waves," I say.

Without wincing or missing a beat, my husband responds with his dry humor, "I already have one prepared." I smile, and the sound of our laughter fills up the car.

About the Author

Alyssa lives in Raleigh, NC with her husband, John, and their dog, Boscoe. Her favorite things in life are hugs, bagels and coffee, spending time in the sunshine, the beach, taking naps, dancing, and laughing with loved ones. She dreams of traveling internationally, learning to play the violin, and becoming fluent in several languages.

As a child, Alyssa would quietly and sweetly talk to anyone. She would abandon her ice cream at the restaurant to go to another table and talk to an elderly person sitting all alone. Conflict pained her. She would jump in between dogs that were fighting, getting bitten in the process. And she was always using the money from her allowance to purchase memberships to various save-the-wildlife foundations.

Because of her gentle and compassionate nature, people with unique life challenges and disabilities have always gravitated toward her. In turn, as she grew up, studying the social sciences and working in settings where she could feel helpful became her natural path. She followed this path into jobs working with inner-city after school programs, nursing homes, home healthcare, and massage therapy. And it is through this journey that she discovered the brokenness within herself.

Despite the challenges of living with Bipolar Disorder and PTSD, Alyssa is committed to reflecting love and light. She explains, "There are days when I have to force myself to get out of bed, and I lack the energy to smile. On days like that, I try to wear something colorful and cheerful that people will notice. Pretty soon, the smiles I receive from other people reflect onto me, and I find myself getting the energy to smile back. I teeter on this edge of laughter and tears. Tears cleanse and laughter heals."

CPSIA information can be obtained
at www.ICGtesting.com
Printed in the USA
BVHW030351010921
615712BV00029B/195